Clean Eating: Best Option for Health

Clean Eating Meal Plan for the Family

By: Nathaniel Grey

TABLE OF CONTENTS

DEDICATION 4

CHAPTER 1- WHAT IS CLEAN EATING? 5

CHAPTER 2- WHAT ARE THE BENEFITS OF EATING CLEAN?..................... 9

CHAPTER 3- HOW TO PLAN GROCERY LISTS AND MEAL PLANS WHEN EATING CLEAN? 13

CHAPTER 4- 10 CLEAN EATING BREAKFAST RECIPES............................ 17

CHAPTER 5- 10 CLEAN EATING LUNCH RECIPES.................................. 26

CHAPTER 6- 10 CLEAN EATING DINNER RECIPES 33

CHAPTER 7- 10 CLEAN EATING DESSERT RECIPES 41

ABOUT THE AUTHOR 49

Nathaniel Grey

PUBLISHERS NOTES

Disclaimer

This publication is intended to provide helpful and informative material. It is not intended to diagnose, treat, cure, or prevent any health problem or condition, nor is intended to replace the advice of a physician. No action should be taken solely on the contents of this book. Always consult your physician or qualified health-care professional on any matters regarding your health and before adopting any suggestions in this book or drawing inferences from it.

The author and publisher specifically disclaim all responsibility for any liability, loss or risk, personal or otherwise, which is incurred as a consequence, directly or indirectly, from the use or application of any contents of this book.

Any and all product names referenced within this book are the trademarks of their respective owners. None of these owners have sponsored, authorized, endorsed, or approved this book.

Always read all information provided by the manufacturers' product labels before using their products. The author and publisher are not responsible for claims made by manufacturers.

© 2013

Manufactured in the United States of America

DEDICATION

This book is dedicated to my Aunt Jessica.

CHAPTER 1 - WHAT IS CLEAN EATING?

It seems as if the world is obsessed with healthy eating fads. From diets to lifestyle changes, many Americans are willing to try anything to raise their energy levels, reduce their weight, or improve their health. While it is great that many people are beginning to focus on nutrition and health it can be confusing to sort through the different dietary options and find the one that best fits your individual needs. However, one of the options definitely worth learning more about and giving a try is clean eating.

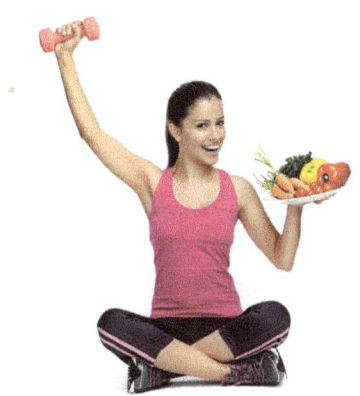

What Clean Eating Isn't

First of all, clean eating is not what most people think of as a diet. The word "diet" has gotten a bad reputation over the past few decades as an extreme change in eating habits that lasts only until a goal is achieved and is not sustainable. Over the past ten years there has been a movement from "dieting" to "lifestyle changes," which are long-term changes in how you relate to and consume

Clean Eating: Best Option for Health

food. Clean eating is definitely a lifestyle change, most beneficial when implemented permanently and not intended only to achieve short-term results. That being said, everything you eat composes your diet, so clean eating is a change in your diet with certain rules and restrictions that you may not be following currently.

Clean eating is similar to many other popular dietary movements including intuitive eating, the raw food movement, and the slow food movement. Even though it is similar to these movements it is not the same. It is a unique approach to food and eating.

What Clean Eating Is

Clean eating is a very basic eating lifestyle in which an individual prioritizes eating food in its most natural state. This commonly means seeking out foods without chemical additives or nutritional supplements. Within the clean eating lifestyle whole foods are given a priority over processed foods. The most common example of this is replacing processed grains such as white flour, with whole grains such as quinoa or whole wheat.

People with the clean eating lifestyle tend to eat more raw vegetables and nuts, and also tend to cook at home more to reduce the amount of fragrances, dyes, and preservatives they consume in prepackaged foods. However, there are prepackaged foods that are suited for the clean eating lifestyle. These foods generally have only one or two ingredients listed on their labels. Another aspect of clean eating is a reduction in the consumption of GMO foods, or foods grown with pesticides.

Though the main focus of clean eating is eating food in its most natural state the clean eating lifestyle often inspires other changes. For example, many people who choose clean eating spend more time cooking their own meals at home and more time consuming those meals than they might have before they made the change to clean eating. Although it is not necessary to cook all of your own meals you will find that you have a greater choice of flavors and textures when you cook at home than you would when you try to follow clean eating while dining out or preparing prepackaged foods.

Some people, instead of spending a lot of time cooking, find themselves eating a diet much higher in raw foods. Another time consuming aspect of clean eating is the growing of vegetables and herbs. Many people following the clean eating lifestyle purchase all of their produce at local shops, but some people find that they become much more aware of where their food is coming from, and pesticides used on non-organic produce, and they find it much more satisfying to grow at least some of their own food.

Benefits of Clean Eating

Clean eating has several benefits. First of all, eating food in its natural state gives an individual a more complete combination of macronutrients and micronutrients. When people begin to rely on nutritional supplements they are often ignoring the fact that nutrients react to one another, and many are not efficiently absorbed or utilized without complementary nutrients. Eating food in its most basic form ensures that you are getting the combination of nutrients that nature intended, resulting in increased overall health. Besides overall health there are some specific benefits that people have experienced from clean eating including maintaining a healthy weight, being less tempted to eat when stressed or depressed, a more regular digestive system, more energy, lower cholesterol levels, and a more regular blood sugar level.

How to Get Started Eating Clean

The first step in transitioning to a clean eating lifestyle is to become aware of your eating habits. Go through your pantry and read the labels on all of your foods. Take note of how much natural food you consume compared to how much processed food. Be aware of preservatives, dyes, and additives. Then, the next time you go shopping try to reduce the amount of processed food you purchase. Follow the rule that if there is anything on the label you cannot pronounce, the food should not be added to your cart. Some people are able to make the transition immediately, cutting out all processed foods from their lives within a week. However, for others it may be a bit of a struggle. It is okay to work at reducing your intake of processed foods as opposed to eliminating it, if that makes you more comfortable.

Some other ways to get started with clean eating are to start a garden or join a community garden, join an organic food co-op, or take a cooking class; each of these activities helps you to become more aware of your eating habits while slightly increasing your intake of unprocessed foods. They are also excellent ways to find friends that share a similar lifestyle as you are trying to achieve. Most importantly, keep in mind that clean eating is not a short-term diet. You cannot expect short-term results when making lifestyle changes for your entire future. For that reason, be patient with yourself and try to have fun as you deepen your relationship with the food you consume.

Chapter 2- What Are the Benefits of Eating Clean?

Eating clean is one of the best things you can do for you and your family. Eating clean is a way of eating healthy foods that do not contain any preservatives. This diet started from the bestselling author Tosca Reno who started the "Eat-Clean Diet" series. Her books focus on eating a healthier way and taking out all of the garbage foods in our diets. Eating clean is eating organic, whole foods, nothing processed, and it shows great results for our body and mind. This chapter will share with you all of the benefits of what eating clean can do for you.

Drops Those Extra Pounds

Eating lean proteins, fresh fruits and vegetables, and drinking plenty of water will help you drop those unwanted pounds. Healthier foods that are not processed give you energy and won't make you feel sluggish. It will help you maintain your exercise regimen or start a new one because you will feel much more energy from eating healthy food rather than that processed junk food in your pantry. Tosca Reno says in her books that if you stay dedicated with the clean eating lifestyle, then you can lose up to three pounds a week. Her philosophy is that eating right is more important than exercise. You have to get the basics down first in order to sustain enough energy to begin a workout program that will help you continue to lose weight. You can exercise like crazy, but if you are eating the wrong kinds of foods, you will not get the results you desire.

Gives You That Healthy Glow

Another great benefit of eating clean is not only burning those calories but also having beautiful skin. Part of eating clean is drinking two to three liters of water a day. Water is such an essential part of our diets because it not only hydrates the body but it flushes out any toxins we may have. Drinking all that water, eating fresh foods, and cutting out all of the processed garbage will make you feel good on both the inside and outside. You will notice a glow in your skin and your hair and nails growing beautifully. Beauty on the outside always starts from within so why not feed yourself the cleanest food possible to get that beautiful glow.

You Get To Eat Six Times A Day!

You will not starve yourself by eating clean. In fact, it is quite the opposite. The Eat Clean diet suggests that you eat six times a day. This means that you will never go hungry and your body will not crave something it shouldn't have. Once your body has gotten used to such healthy food, you will no longer get those cravings for fast food. It may even make your stomach turn by looking at it knowing how bad it can make your body feel.

You Get To Eat Delicious Food

Eating clean means that you get to eat the most delicious and healthiest food around. No prepackaged, tiny, calorie counting meals sent to your door that looks scary. Remember that eating clean means that you get to shop for the freshest foods possible. Once you get use to eating such fresh and healthy foods, you will not want to go back to foods with added chemicals in them ever again. And let's be honest here, unprocessed food tastes way better than the processed garbage.

What Is Good For the Body Is Also Good For the Mind

Not only will you lose weight, gain energy, and eat delicious meals, but eating clean will also help you focus. Eating clean for breakfast will give you a jump start on your day and it won't have you feeling tired in an hour. Also, getting your children to eat a clean breakfast can help them stay focused in school. Foods on our market shelves today that are geared towards children are loaded with chemicals and dyes that can have a major effect on our children's behavior throughout the day.

It Can Save You Money

You may wonder how buying organic and unprocessed foods at your local farmers market or grocery store can actually save you money. It will save you money in the long run because your family will enjoy the taste of such quality foods that you will never let any of it go to waste. We often purchase frozen foods and packaged processed foods that are affordable; however, many times they get thrown out because the quality of the food is not very good. Your family will push those foods to the side and eventually you throw them away because no one ate them. Having fresh and healthy foods in your house available for your family is worth spending your money on.

Recipes Galore!

The best part about eating clean is all of the recipes available to you. There are many websites and cookbooks that focus on eating clean and healthy. If you enjoy cooking, then you will really love making meals the eating clean way. No need to worry about this diet not having enough flavors in your meals. You will notice how much more flavor eating clean has compared to eating meals with processed foods.

It's Easy!

Clean Eating: Best Option for Health

Some people may think that eating clean looks complicated but it really is simple. Once you know what to look out for and purchase at the grocery store, it will get much easier. Make a list for every grocery trip, it will help you stay focused on the things that you need and shop for whole grains, fresh fruits, vegetables, healthy proteins and fats. Avoid any foods with added sugars, salt, and refined grains. You will love how great the food tastes and be amazed at how much weight you will lose without ever having to count any calories! Once you embrace these healthy new foods and see all of the benefits, changing your lifestyle will be easy!

Chapter 3- How to Plan Grocery Lists and Meal Plans When Eating Clean?

It's sometimes required in maintaining your vitality, youthfulness, and energy to make the transition to clean eating. If you want the best out of life, you must start with taking care of yourself as a whole. From eating right, exercising, getting enough rest, routine doctor visits, etc., it's no getting around improving and maintaining yourself holistically. With that being said, organization comes into play. You must organize your day accordingly, to accomplish your daily tasks without over exhaustion, and in order to do the required things necessary in taking care of yourself. As a matter of fact, you must also set some time every now and then, to do clean eating, that is also required for a holistic well being.

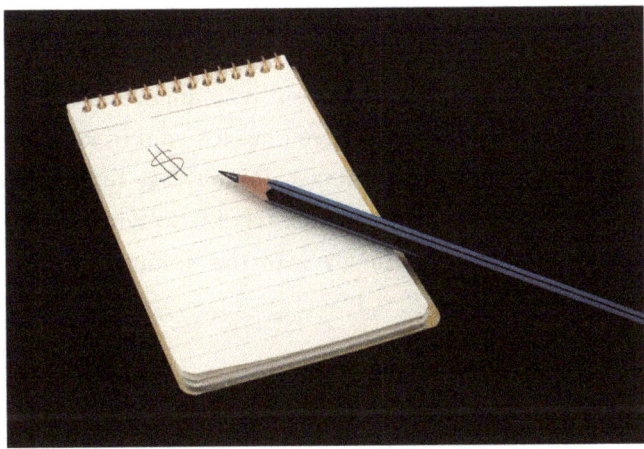

Clean eating is like a partial fast that has so many health benefits. With it, your organs and mental capabilities are tremendously improved. Also, you will gain a burst of energy, as you go from day to day, when undergoing the clean eating process. You will eliminate stress from your life, and as we all know, stress is a silent killer. Toxins are also expelled from the body, you'll have a better aspect in life, and your overall condition will improved significantly. Let's face it--this is crucial for your whole well being.

In undergoing the clean eating process, certain steps and organizing must be adhered to. For one, you must set out a plan. Take some time out to brainstorm all that needs to be done, and all that you need from the grocery store for your clean eating. This will take some ample time, and so, this is not a time to rush through this process. It's vital to evaluate and think thoroughly on all that you must do and buy for the success of this period.

Once that is done, you should make a "To Do" list and a grocery list if you don't have all the types of food available for the clean eating. As a matter of fact, it may be best to make a list while you brainstorm, to ensure that you don't forget anything. Sure with brainstorming, the list will be a rough draft, but at least you are writing things down as you brainstorm, which will reduce your chances of forgetting important tasks and/or groceries.

Once that is completed, the next step is to adhere to the "To Do" List and the grocery list, if you have one. It's vital to keep in mind, the length of time for this partial fast. The average time to undergo this process is between two to three weeks. So with this in mind, you must plan things accordingly with the amount of food, your budget, and other tasks.

While grocery shopping, you must keep in mind your budget. Sometimes, the more healthier and lean food items are the most expensive. However, catching sales, using coupons, checking clearance racks, and going to dollar store outlets can contribute to your budget drastically. With utilizing most to all of these techniques, you will be able to save big, and purchase everything on your list and possibly more.

Next, to have a clean eating period, you need to have whole grains, lean meats (or for some, no meat at all, and if that's the case, you must make sure to consume the adequate amount of protein). Low sodium foods, gluten free foods for some who elects this, and a variety of fruits and vegetables are also needed. Of course, it's important to have these food choices in your regular diet too, for great nutrition value. However, it's even more important during the clean eating period.

Normally, the prices of different whole grains like different types of pasta and bread are very reasonable. However if you find that you need to lower the price of whole grains even further, coupons can be a great choice. Also, you can check for day old bread from the bakery, and even the clearance racks may have some assortment of whole grains.

Another great food item that is very low in cost but very high in nutritional value is a different array of beans. Beans are very affordable. The costs of beans can range from pennies off of a dollar to about $2.00 per pack. And these packs that are worth about $2.00 are really huge in quantity. So, getting a variety of shapes, sizes, and brands of beans can be quite helpful with the nutritional value. Additionally, with beans, you can eat them as a side dish, or use them in stews, soups, and casseroles, which will go a long way for your budget, and time for cooking. With beans being used in stews, soups, or casseroles, you can have leftovers for a few days.

With fruits and veggies, you can check the farmer's market. They always have great products at great prices. Otherwise, you can sometimes catch sales, or even get coupons on these items.

Some things are important to keep in mind, when shopping for fruits and vegetables. For one thing, you must be aware that the shelf life for fruits and vegetables are very limited. So, you must get a limited amount at a time. Besides, even though eating plenty of fruit and vegetables is important, you can overeat these things, which can cause huge problems for your digestive system. Another thing to keep in mind concerning fruits and vegetables is that it's important to know how to pick them. For vegetables, make sure to get some without brown, withering edges. For fruits, the potency of the smell and the weight of the fruit in some cases, indicate the great level of sweetness/ripeness of the fruit. And lastly, if you get can fruits and vegetables, make sure to notice the ingredients, make sure there's no dent in the can, and check the expiration dates.

When you apply these techniques properly, you will successfully be on your way to a better, healthier you.

Chapter 4- 10 Clean Eating Breakfast Recipes

Cheesy Potato Frittata

Ingredients

2 ounce shredded low-fat sharp cheddar cheese
1 clove minced garlic
1½ cups yellow onion, diced
1 teaspoon safflower oil
½ teaspoon sea salt, divided
½ teaspoon black pepper (fresh ground)
1 tablespoon fresh thyme (chopped)
¼ cup finely fresh parsley (chopped)
2 tablespoon skim milk
1 large egg plus 6 egg whites
8 new potatoes, scrubbed well and cut into 1/2-inch cubes
¼ cup green onion, finely chopped (optional)
½ cup low-fat sour cream (optional)

Directions

On medium high heat, boil 2 cups water and then put in the potatoes and let water come to a boil. Lower the heat and let simmer until tender (twelve minutes). Drain and put to the side.

In a bowl, whisk ¼ teaspoon salt, pepper, thyme, parsley, milk, egg whites and egg then set aside.

In a mid-sized skillet to heat some oil. Put in the onion and stir frequently, until the edges start to brown (about six minutes). Put in the garlic and keep stirring for another fifteen seconds. Put the potatoes in and combine well. Turn down heat to. Whisk egg mixture gently and pour evenly on top of potato mix. Cover and cook until the mix is almost set (twelve minutes). Take skillet off heat and mix in the rest of the cheddar and 1/4 teaspoon salt. Cover and leave sit for fifteen minutes. Get the frittata and cut 4 wedges. On top of these wedges put some green onions and sour cream.

Breakfast Quinoa

Ingredients

1 teaspoon cinnamon, optional
⅔ cup raisins or chocolate chips, optional
⅛ teaspoon pure Stevia extract or ¼ cup sweetener of choice
1 teaspoon pure vanilla extract
4 cups milk of choice
2½ cups water
1 teaspoon salt
1 cup raw quinoa

Directions

Get a fine mesh strainer and rinse the quinoa in it. After draining mix the quinoa with some water and salt and let come to a boil. Cover and cook until the quinoa is fluffy and light (twenty minutes on low heat). Put in milk, cinnamon and raisins (optional) and let come to a boil. Turn down heat and keep cooking for another thirty minutes. Remember to stir often. The mixture should be nice and thick. After turning heat off put in sweetener and vanilla.

Apple Cinnamon Quinoa Bites

Ingredients

2 lightly beaten eggs

Nathaniel Grey

1 cup apples (chopped)
1 tablespoon maple syrup
1 tablespoon sugar (granulated)
3 tablespoons sugar (brown)
½ teaspoon nutmeg
½ teaspoon cinnamon
1 cup quick oats
1 cup cooked quinoa

Directions

Preheat the oven to 350 degrees.

In a big bowl add the quick oats and the quinoa. In another bowl mix the sugars, nutmeg, and cinnamon. Put the spice mix in the oats and quinoa mix. Put in eggs, apples and maple syrup and mix well. Use some olive oil to grease a small muffin pan.

Put 1 teaspoon of the mix in each slot and place in oven to bake for approximately twenty minutes.

Honey Cloud Pancakes

Ingredients

Honey
Soft fruits
1 tablespoon of butter
A dash of vanilla extract
2 teaspoon of honey
A pinch of salt
¼ cup of four
¼ cup of milk (warmed)
1 egg white and 1 large egg

Directions

Heat the oven to 350 degrees Fahrenheit. Place a small frying pan (ove n proof) in oven to heat.

Whisk egg white until peaks start to form and in another bowl mix an egg with vanilla, honey, salt and flour. Whisk the warm milk in. Use a metal spoon to fold the egg white gently into the batter. In the pan melt the butter then put in the batter and let cook for approximately five minutes. Put the fruit on the top and place in oven until it has a golden color (7 minutes).

Use the rest of the honey to drizzle on top.

Super Foods Smoothie

Ingredients

1 cup crushed ice
½ cup pure pomegranate juice
1 cup unsweetened green tea (chilled)
½ cup plain Greek Yogurt, 0% fat
½ inch slice Fresh ginger root
1 cup unsweetened frozen berries
1 small sliced frozen banana
1 cup loosely packed baby spinach (organic)

Directions

Mix all the ingredients in a blender and combine until the texture is smooth. If you prefer a thinner consistency add more green tea.

Clean Sticky Buns

Ingredients

Nathaniel Grey

1 tablespoon cinnamon (ground)
1/4 cup unsalted pecans (chopped)
1/2 teaspoon Sucanat
1 teaspoon raw honey
1/4 cup pure maple syrup
3 tablespoons organic unsalted butter, divided
2 teaspoons quick-rise active dry yeast
2 teaspoons plus 2 tablespoon organic evaporated cane juice, divided
1/4 teaspoon fine sea salt
2 cups flour, plus more for rolling
Cooking spray or Olive oil

Directions

Spray a big bowl with the cooking spray and put to one side. Mix flour and salt in food processor.

Mix cane juice and half cup lukewarm water in a 1 cup measure then add yeast and keep stirring until combined. Let sit until foamy (approximately 5 minutes) then turn on the food processor and add the yeast mix and let pulse for about two minutes. As soon as dough starts to form let pulse for another minute. Place the dough in a bowl and turn it so it is coated thoroughly. Use a plastic wrap to cover it and leave dough to rise to double its size (1 hour).

Use cooking spray to coat a square baking pan (8 inch). In a pot or saucepan, melt one and a half tablespoons butter. Place the butter in the baking pan. Put in maple syrup and use spoon to combine mix and to coat the bottom of the pan thoroughly. Drizzle on honey and sprinkle with pecans and Sucanat and put to one side.

Flour rolling surface lightly and then roll the dough into a rectangle (8 x 12). Spread the rest of the butter on top of the dough and then sprinkle on cinnamon and cane juice. Roll the dough lengthwise, ensuring that you pinch the edge to prevent dough from unrolling. Cut into twelve pieces and then place them in the baking pan with the flat side down. Leave enough space between them so they are not touching. Use plastic wrap to cover and leave at room temperature to rise to double its size (approximately forty five minutes).

Preheat the oven to 375°F. Remove the plastic wrap from the pan and place in the oven and let bake for about twenty five minutes until golden. Take out of the oven and place buns on a big plate and serve.

Apple Stuffed French Toast

Ingredients

Apples:

1 teaspoon pure maple syrup
1 teaspoon vanilla extract
1/2 teaspoon cinnamon (ground)
2 teaspoons light flavored oil such as grape seed or safflower
2 thinly sliced medium tart apples

Toast:

Maple syrup for topping
8 slices of whole grain bread
1/4 of the cooked apples
1/2 teaspoon allspice
3 whole eggs
2 cups almond milk (unsweetened)

Directions

In a mid- sized pot mix the vanilla, cinnamon, oil and apples. Cook on low heat until the apples are soft (twenty minutes). in a big mixing bowl whisk the allspice, eggs and almond milk.

Pour a bit of the milk mix into a baking dish (9 x 13) then put a layer of bread in the pan and put a quarter of the bread filling on the top. Put another layer of bread and add some more liquid. After about a minute flip the bread. Replace any stuffing that falls out. Ensure the bread gets soaked on both sides. Bake in an oven that has been heated to 350 degrees Fahrenheit for about twenty five minutes. The bread should be brown on top. When done, let cool then pour some maple syrup on top.

Banana Breakfast Doughnuts

Ingredients

2 cups mashed banana (tightly-packed)
1 Stevia packet
1½ tablespoon lemon juice
½ cup pure maple or agave syrup
1½ teaspoon pure vanilla extract
2 tablespoons of milk
¼ cup oil
¾ teaspoon salt
¾ teaspoon baking powder
½ teaspoon cinnamon
1 teaspoon baking soda
2 cups flour
Optional: shredded coconut, walnuts or chocolate chips

Directions

Preheat oven to 350 Fahrenheit. In a bowl combine the dry ingredients. Combine the wet ingredients in another bowl and then use hand to combine the ingredients. When fully combined, spoon the mix into a muffin pan that has been greased. Place in oven for approximately thirty five minutes.

Raisin & Oatmeal Raisin Cookies

Ingredients

1 packet Stevia
1/16 teaspoon salt
3 tablespoon raisins (chocolate chips and dried fruit can be used as well)
½ teaspoon pure vanilla extract
¼ teaspoon cinnamon
¼ cup nut butter
½ cup over- ripe mashed banana or applesauce
½ cup rolled oats

Directions

Preheat oven to 350 degrees Fahrenheit. Crush the nut butter with the applesauce or banana. Put in the remaining ingredients and combine. Form the cookies and place in oven to bake for approximately fourteen minutes.

Breakfast Pizza

Ingredients

A few handfuls of raisins, walnuts, chopped apples, chocolate chips or raspberries
Extracts or spices or extracts (if desired)
⅛ teaspoon salt
2 tablespoon coconut oil or applesauce
½ cup milk, juice or water

Nathaniel Grey
2 Stevia packets
1 teaspoon baking powder
½ cup pastry flour (whole-wheat)

Directions

Combine all the ingredients and place them in a pan that is greased. Cook in a cold oven for approximately ten minutes at 420 degrees Fahrenheit. Add toppings and serve.

CHAPTER 5- 10 CLEAN EATING LUNCH RECIPES

Clean eating is a healthy alternative to fast food, processed food and foods that simply are not feeding the body in the best possible manner. Lunchtime tends to be the one meal where people opt for fast over healthy; however, clean eating lunch recipes can be simple, fast and nutritious so one can ditch that drive through window once and for all.

Chicken and Lettuce Wraps

Ingredients

Thinly sliced grilled or broiled chicken
Romaine lettuce
Sliced tomatoes
Thinly sliced red onion
Red wine vinegar
Extra virgin olive oil

Directions

Place a full size, outer leaf of lettuce on a plate and lay flat. Layer the sliced chicken, tomatoes and red onion on top of the chicken. Drizzle the olive oil and red wine vinegar on top to taste. Roll the lettuce to wrap and secure with a toothpick.

Chopped Salad

Ingredients

Baby green lettuce mix
Red onion

Cucumbers
Green bell pepper
Red bell pepper
Drained chickpeas
Oregano
Salt and pepper
Greek nonfat yogurt
Lemon juice
Dill
Minced garlic

Directions

Chop all vegetables in to small pieces of equal size and place in a bowl off to the side. Whisk together the dressing by combining the Greek yogurt, lemon juice, dill and garlic. Blend the dressing until smooth and pour over top of the chopped vegetables. Sprinkle a little oregano, salt and pepper over top to taste.

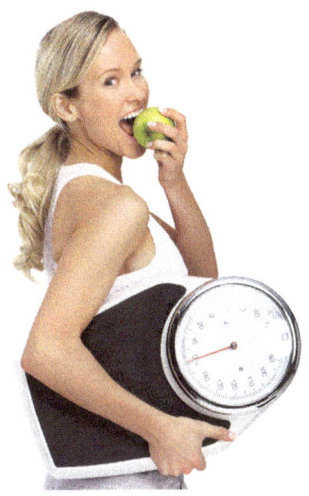

Egg White Omelet

Ingredients

Egg whites
Low or no fat cheddar cheese, shredded
Diced green peppers and onions
Nonfat cooking spray

Directions

In a small bowl whisk the egg whites until fluffy. Spray a pan with cooking spray and allow to heat up. Pour the egg mixture in and allow to cook for three to five minutes and then place the diced peppers, onions and shredded cheese on top. Fold in half so the vegetables and cheese are covered. Cook one to two more minutes, flip and then cook until the cheese is melted.

Bibb Lettuce Boats

Ingredients

Whole head of Bibb lettuce
Canned tuna or chicken
Diced red onion
Fresh mozzarella or blue cheese
Extra virgin olive oil
Balsamic vinegar
Salt and pepper

Directions

Remove the core of the lettuce to create a Bibb lettuce cup. Inside of the lettuce layer the drained chicken or tuna, onion and cheese. Drizzle the olive oil and balsamic vinegar over top and season to taste with the salt and pepper.

Flaked Tuna Salad

Albacore tuna in water, drained
Diced sweet onion
Diced celery
Celery seed
Lemon juice
Salt and pepper

Directions

In a small bowl, mix together the tuna, onion, celery and celery seed until well blended. Drizzle lemon juice on top and mix again until well incorporated throughout. Season with salt and pepper to taste. This can be eaten alone or on top of lettuce or whole wheat pita bread.

Nuts and Berries Salad

Ingredients

Assortment of nuts (almonds, walnuts, pecans and peanuts)
Chopped baby greens
Dried berries (cranberries, blueberries, blackberries and strawberries)
Extra virgin olive oil
Balsamic vinegar

Directions

Toss the nuts and berries with the olive oil and balsamic vinegar until all are coated well. Place the nuts and berries mixture on top of fresh baby greens for a sweet and savory salad. Additional chopped up vegetables can be added if on hand.

Protein Shake

Protein powder
Banana
Strawberries
Ice cubes
Soy or almond milk
Vanilla extract

Directions

In a blender combine all ingredients and pulsated until the ice cubes have been broken in to small pieces. Continue blending until smooth and thick. More protein powder can be added for extra thickness and alternate fruits can be used based on what is in season.

Chickpea Salad

Ingredients

Canned chickpeas, drained
Fresh chopped dill
Finely diced red onion
Finely diced cucumber
Finely diced eggplant
Finely diced roasted red peppers (drained)
Balsamic vinegar

Directions

In a small bowl mix all ingredients and add balsamic vinegar to taste. In addition, salt and pepper can be used to season if desired. The salad can be eaten alone, with a wide of fresh pits chips or on top of chopped baby greens or spinach.

Hummus and Pita Chips

Nathaniel Grey
Ingredients

Canned chickpeas, drained
Tahini
Lemon juice
Minced fresh garlic
Finely minced sweet onion
Chopped roasted red peppers, drained
Salt and pepper
Oregano
Pita bread
Extra virgin olive oil

Directions

In a blender combine drained chickpeas, tahini, lemon juice, garlic, onion, roasted red peppers, salt, pepper and oregano. Blend well until the consistency is thick and smooth. A small drizzle of olive oil may be needed to make the hummus smooth and creamy. Slice the pita bread in to triangles and heat a small amount of olive oil in a pan. Heat and crisp the pita bread for two minutes per side and place on paper towels to drain. Season pita chips with salt, pepper and oregano for added flavor.

Stir Fry

Cooked protein (lean fish, chicken or tofu)
Low sodium soy sauce
Sliced vegetables (onions, snap peas, carrots, broccoli, bok choy, sprouts, mushrooms, red bell peppers, etc.)

Directions

In a sauté pan place one-half inch of soy sauce and add all other ingredients. Bring the mixture to a high heat and cover for five

Clean Eating: Best Option for Health

minutes to partially cook the vegetables. Lower the heat and cook, covered, for an additional ten minutes or until the vegetables are tender. Splash a little extra soy sauce on top before serving.

CHAPTER 6- 10 CLEAN EATING DINNER RECIPES

Eating healthy doesn't have to be an activity reserved for January 1. Nor does it have to require a lot of effort and money. Eating clean and balancing a healthy lifestyle is a very important part of maintaining life longevity. Learning about basic nutrition and focusing on healthy eating habits will improve your immune system, boost your energy levels, and keep you on track for reduced health risks.

Most people struggle with preparing a clean mean for dinner. After a long day at work, the last thing on your mind is preparing and cooking a fresh and healthy meal. Instead, most deviate to the nearest drive through, to satisfy their hunger by a quick fix. In attempts to avoid that fast food detour, below are 10 clean dinner recipes to try.

If you enjoy fresh fish, then we recommend you indulge in this recipe.

Salmon

Ingredients

1 pound salmon filet
2 tablespoons olive oil
1 TABLESPOON dill
1 tablespoon lemon juice
4 basil leaves
1 tablespoon paprika
1 cedar plank soaked for one hour
Pepper to taste

Directions

Preheat your over to 425.

Drizzle olive oil and lemon juice on the pink side. Pour the dill and paprika on top. Place basil over the seasoning

Place pink side of salmon down on the cedar plank. Pour the other tablespoon. of olive oil on the skin. Bake for 15 to 20 minutes. Sprinkle with pepper to taste

Healthy Caprese Salad

Ingredients

2 tablespoons olive oil
1 large red tomato
1 large yellow tomato
1 red onion diced
4 chopped basil leaves
Pepper to taste

Directions

Cut both the red and yellow tomatoes into bite sized slices

Place into a bowl. Top them with the olive oil. Sprinkle the basil leaves in and mix and then toss in the onions

Add pepper to taste

Turkey Fresh Fajitas

Ingredients

Guacamole (premade or your own version)

2 garlic cloves
4 teaspoon olive oil
2 tablespoons lime juice
1 teaspoon ground cumin
1 teaspoon chili powder
1 red bell pepper
1 onion
1½ lbs turkey, cut into thin slices
1 bunch of scallions, chopped
¼ cup fresh cilantro

Directions

In a large bowl, prepare the olive oil, chopped garlic, lime, cumin and chili powder. Add the sliced turkey and mix thoroughly. Chill for 2 hours.

Get a skillet and heat up the remaining 2 tablespoon. of olive oil. Put in onion and peppers into the skillet. Add the turkey and cook for about 10 minutes, constantly stirring the mixture. Top with scallions and cilantro. Add guacamole.

Below are a few beef recipes that are healthy without sacrificing much of the flavor.

Pot Roast for Clean Eating

Ingredients

1 teaspoon chili powder
1 teaspoon ground cumin
1 teaspoon cayenne pepper
1 teaspoon oregano
1 teaspoon paprika
2 lb chuck roast

Clean Eating: Best Option for Health

1 C red wine
1 C chicken broth (low sodium)
1 tablespoon olive oil
4 celery stalks, cut into bite size pieces
4 carrots, cut into bite sized pieces
1 onion, cut into eight pieces

Directions

Combine all dry spices into a large cooking bowl, take the roast and place it into the bowl, and ensure the roast is fully covered with the seasoning on all sides. In a deep pot, heat the olive oil.

Brown the seasoned roast for 8-9 minutes. Turn to make sure it cooks evenly and then add vegetables and sauté.

Add the broth and the red wine and bring to a boil. Reduce heat and cover. Let simmer for 2 and a half hours, stirring every 20 minutes

Carne Asada

Ingredients

2 lbs beef flank
1 jalapeño
1 teaspoon ground cumin
2 tablespoons olive oil
2 tablespoons cilantro
1 teaspoon lime juice

Directions

Combine all ingredients (except the beef) into a container. Place beef on a flat plate. Pour ingredients over the steak

Cool for 2 hours. You can either BBQ this, grill this on your stove top, or broil it. If you decide to broil this, do so for 10 minutes, turning it each 5 minutes. For those of you who enjoy lighter meat, here are some recipes for great tasting poultry!

Cashew & Coconut Chicken

Ingredients

4 skinless and boneless breasts of chicken (tenderized)
1 C coconut curry
¼ C cashews
1 scallion

Directions

Mix the curry with the chicken and chill for 2 hours. Set your oven to the broil setting. Cook for 20 minutes, and turn it every 10 minutes. Remove from the broiler and top with chopped scallions and cashews.

Northern Chicken Breasts

Ingredients

1 tablespoon parsley, chopped finely
2 tablespoon olive oil
1 tablespoon tarragon, chopped finely
4 bone-in breasts of chicken
2 cup chicken broth (low sodium)
Black pepper to taste
1 tomato finely diced
8oz sliced mushrooms
1 shallot, finely diced

Directions

Preheat your over to 425 degrees. Heat olive oil over stove in a skillet and add chicken breasts and top the chicken breasts with the black pepper. Cover this and cook for 5 minutes per side.

Remove chicken from the heat, and set aside. Place mushrooms in the pan and cook then for around 10 minutes

Add the broth with the tomatoes and bring this to a boil. Once boiling, reduce to simmer for 5 minutes. Place chicken back into the skillet, cover and bake for roughly 20 minutes or until chicken is fully cooked.

Remove and top with parsley and tarragon

Chicken Marsala

Eating clean doesn't mean you have to toss old favorite recipes and family dishes. It simply means that you just need to revise the ingredients, so you make it a "healthy" version of your favorite dish

Ingredients

4 skinless and boneless breasts of chicken
1 cup chopped mushrooms
2 tablespoons olive oil
1 shallot chopped finely
½ teaspoon oregano
½ C Marsala red wine
½ chicken broth (reduced sodium)

Directions

In a skillet, heat the olive oil

Add the 4 chicken breasts and cook for about 10 minutes, rotating at 5 minutes. Remove from the skillet and cover with foil. Add 1 cup mushrooms and cook for 5 minutes. Add the shallot and cook another minute

Slowly pour in the chicken broth and wine, and bring to a nice boil. Reduce heat. Simmer the mixture for 20 minutes

Add the chicken back into the skillet and top with oregano and let cook for 5 minutes

For those of you who enjoy a more "rare" type of meat, here is a recipe for you!

Juicy Veal

Ingredients

4 cuts of veal
2 tablespoons olive oil
¼ cup parsley, finely chopped
1 cup cremini mushrooms
1 shallot, chopped

Directions

Heat only one tablespoon. in skillet, place veal into skillet and let cook for 4 minutes, turning it every 2 minutes.

Place the veal on a plate covered in paper towels to dry off. Add the other tablespoon. of olive oil to the skillet along with the mushrooms and shallot. Cook for about 5 minutes. Add the broth and boil for a minute. Reduce heat and slowly and carefully add the veal to the skillet and cook for one minute. Top with parsley

BBQ Bison Ribs

Dare to try a more protein packed meat? Then try the recipe below and enjoy!

Ingredients

12 Bison ribs
1 cup Raspberry BBQ sauce
1 teaspoon rosemary
2 garlic cloves, chopped very finely
1 teaspoon thyme, dried
2 bay leaves
1 teaspoon basil

Directions

Separate each of the 12 ribs individually. In a pot, warm up 4 quarts of water and add the dry spices and the garlic into a mixing bowl. Add spices into the heated water. Bring the water to a boil and slowly and carefully add in the ribs and reduce to a simmer and cook for 10 minutes.

Take ribs out of pot and place into a large mixing bowl. Turn on your BBQ to a medium heat. Take the raspberry BBQ sauce and generously brush onto the ribs. Place ribs on your BBQ and cook for 15 minutes and enjoy!

As you have noticed by now, we have substituted olive oil in all of these recipes in lieu of butter. This minor change make a vast difference in helping you obtain your clean eating goals. We hope that you enjoy the recipes we have provided to you for your clean eating dinner recipes. They are fairly easy to make, with minimal ingredients, and many fresh ingredients.

Chapter 7- 10 Clean Eating Dessert Recipes

Chocolate & Zucchini Muffins

Ingredients

¼ cup chocolate chips
1 teaspoon cinnamon
2 teaspoon baking soda
½ teaspoon salt
½ cup cocoa powder
¼ cup ground flax seed
2 cups whole wheat flour
2 cups chopped up zucchini
1 teaspoon vanilla
¾ cup plain yogurt
1 banana (mashed)
2 egg whites and 1 egg
¼ cup coconut oil
¼ cup molasses
⅓ cup honey

Directions

Preheat the oven to 375 degrees. Take the zucchini and shred it then combine the zucchini and wet ingredients. Mix the cinnamon, baking soda, salt, cocoa powder, ground flaxseed and flour in another bowl. Add to the wet mix and combine well. Put in the chocolate chips and mix.

Use oil to coat the muffin tin and fill each slot half way. Place in oven for approximately twenty minutes to bake.

Clean Eating: Best Option for Health

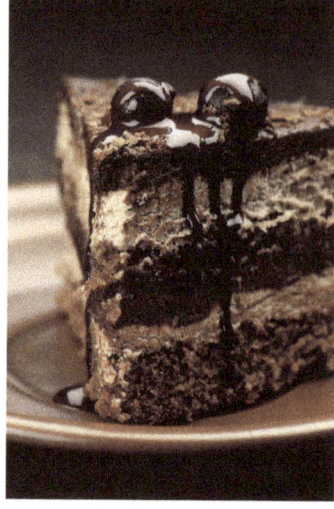

Special Mug Cake

Ingredients

¾ tablespoon mashed-up banana
2 tablespoon milk
1 packet of truvia
1 pinch salt
¼ teaspoon baking powder
1 teaspoon cocoa powder
2 tablespoon wheat flour

Directions

In a mug combine all the dry ingredients. Put in the milk and place in the microwave for sixty seconds.

Chocolate Peanut Butter Cake

Ingredients

1 teaspoon baking powder

Nathaniel Grey

3 tablespoon peanut flour
3 tablespoon oat flour
Unsweetened cocoa powder
4 packets of truvia
¼ cup applesauce (unsweetened)
⅓ cup almond milk
1 tablespoon flaxseed (ground)
⅛ teaspoon salt

Directions

Mix the almond milk and ground flaxseed. Add the salt, truvia and applesauce and mix then out in the peanut flour, oat flour and cocoa powder. Mix in the baking powder. Place the batter in a baking dish (shallow) and place in the microwave for approximately five minutes.

Black Bean Brownies

Ingredients

½ cup to ⅔ cup chocolate chips
½ teaspoon baking powder
2 teaspoon vanilla extract
¼ cup coconut oil
2 tablespoon sugar (or replace with extra 1/2 cup maple syrup)
⅓ cup maple syrup
¼ teaspoon salt
½ cup quick oats
2 tablespoon cocoa powder
1½ cups black beans

Directions

Preheat the oven to 350 degrees Fahrenheit. Mix all of the ingredients in a food processor, except the chips and combine until texture is smooth. Mix in the chips and pour mixture in a baking dish (8 x 8). Let brownies bake for approximately eighteen minutes.

Almond Honey Cookies

Ingredients

4 egg whites
¾ cup honey
1½ cups ground almonds

Directions

In a big bowl, beat the egg whites until the peaks form. In a next bowl combine the honey and almonds and then scoop this into the egg whites and fold to combine. Use a teaspoon to place lumps on some parchment paper. Place in oven to bake for approximately fifteen minutes.

Grandma's Gingerbread Cookies

Ingredients

2 teaspoon vanilla extract
4 tablespoon applesauce
¼ teaspoon nutmeg
¼ teaspoon cloves
2 teaspoon cinnamon
1 egg
¾ tablespoon ginger
¼ teaspoon salt
¾ teaspoon baking soda
1½ teaspoon baking powder

Nathaniel Grey
¼ cup molasses
1 tablespoon and ⅓ cup maple syrup
3 cups flour

Directions

In a bowl mix the dry ingredients. In a next bowl mix all mix all the wet ingredients then add to the dry and mix to combine. Take the dough out of the bowl and cut into equal parts. Use plastic to wrap the dough and place in the refrigerator for a minimum of two hours.

Preheat the oven to 350 degrees Fahrenheit. Remove the dough from the refrigerator and roll out dough until it is a ¼ inch thick. Cut various shapes in dough and place them on a lined baking sheet. Let the cookies bake for about 8 minutes.

Olivia's Oatmeal Muffins

Ingredients

½ cup chocolate chips
½ teaspoon cinnamon
½ teaspoon salt
1 teaspoon baking powder
½ cup sugar
1½ cup spelt flour
1 cup rolled oats
3 tablespoon coconut oil
1 cup mashed banana
½ cup applesauce
2 teaspoon vanilla extract
1½ tablespoon apple cider vinegar
1 cup milk

Directions

Preheat the oven to 400 degrees. Get fifteen muffin tins and put liners in them. Combine the last coconut oil, mashed banana, applesauce, vanilla extract, apple cider vinegar and milk in a bowl. Combine the remaining ingredients in another bowl. Fold wet ingredients in to the dry and combine. Place mixture in muffin tins and place in oven to bake for approximately eighteen minutes.

Pistachio Truffles

Ingredients

Filling:

¼ teaspoon sea salt
1 tablespoon water
1 teaspoon ground vanilla bean or extract
8 medjool dates
1 cup unsalted pistachios

Chocolate Coating

1 tablespoon coconut oil
¼ cup milk
½ cup chocolate chips

Directions

Filling:

Coarsely ground pistachios in food processor and put the rest of the ingredients in and pulse until dough begins to form. Form balls with the dough and place on a plate lined with parchment and place in freezer for about half an hour.

Chocolate Coating:

Melt the milk, coconut milk and chocolate in a double boiler. Mix until the consistency is thin and smooth. Take the balls of dough out of the freezer. Place balls in the chocolate mix and use forks to coat thoroughly and place them back on the plate. As soon as all the balls are coated, place them back in the freezer for another half an hour.

Blackberry Yogurt Popsicles

Ingredients

1 teaspoon vanilla extract
¼ cup honey
1 cup frozen blackberries
2 cups non fat yogurt

Directions

In a tall blending pitcher place the ingredients and combine until smooth. Place in Popsicle molds and place in refrigerator to freeze.

Lemon Blueberry Yogurt Cake

Ingredients

⅓ cup extra blueberries
1 cup blueberries
2 extra tablespoon sugar
1 teaspoon salt
4 teaspoon baking powder
⅔ cups sugar
2 cups all purpose flour
3 tablespoon coconut oil

1 teaspoon vanilla extract
1½ tablespoon lemon zest
1 tablespoon ground flax
½ cup plain yogurt
¼ cup lemon juice
¾ cup milk

Directions

Grease a baking pan (9½ inches) and preheat the oven to 350 degrees Fahrenheit. Mix the milk, lemon juice, plain yogurt, ground flax, lemon zest, vanilla extract and coconut oil and put to one side. Mix the rest of the ingredients (except the blueberries) in another bowl. Combine the dry and wet ingredients. Place the batter in the greased pan and spread the blueberries on top. Place in oven for approximately fifty minutes. When done remove from oven and let cool before taking cake out of the pan.

Nathaniel Grey

ABOUT THE AUTHOR

Nathaniel Grey's mother always told him that it was better if he ate healthy foods in the long run. He would have fewer visits to the doctor and he would feel better overall. He kept this in mind and spent all of his time making sure that he was eating properly as an adult. Of course a sweet treat every now and then did not hurt at all.

When he went off to university he found a similar group of friends that had the same set of principles instilled in them. Together they decided to spread the word on being healthy.

www.ingramcontent.com/pod-product-compliance
Ingram Content Group UK Ltd.
Pitfield, Milton Keynes, MK11 3LW, UK
UKHW022120230426
12048UKWH00010BA/617